The Truth About Carbs:

Know How To Eat The Exact Amount Of Carbs To Melt Fat,
Look Great Naked, And Stay Lean All Year

Introduction

I want to thank you and congratulate you for downloading the book, *"The Truth About Carbs: Know How To Eat The Exact Amount Of Carbs To Melt Fat, Look Great Naked, And Stay Lean All Year."*

So many have tried countless dieting regimes — detox, vegan, Paleo, South Beach, etc. — but many had not yet met success in terms of weight loss and achieving a leaner, slimmer figure. What could be the problem? While the ultimate goal is to lose weight, some people have trouble losing *fat*. This book is aimed toward those dieters and anyone who wants to learn how to melt fat and stay lean, by focusing on the ever-elusive, ever-controversial *carbohydrates*.

This book will teach you the *truth* about carbs and how you can deal with this molecule. You don't have to *completely eliminate* carbs and say goodbye to your favorite food groups (never say goodbye to pastries or pasta!). You will learn how to eat carbs the proper way — for the benefit of your health and the success of your fat-loss endeavor.

Thanks again for downloading this book, I hope you enjoy it!

Table of Contents

Chapter 1: All About Carbs

Over the years, there have been mixed opinions and reactions about carbohydrates, or simply, *carbs*. The controversy about carbs is similar to sugar. One study would tell you that you that sugar is vital and does not cause any *fat gain*. Then another study would pop up and tell the dieting world that sugar is practically poisonous to the body: It causes diseases, makes you accumulate fat, and ultimately harms your health.

What is the truth about these claims? Nobody can tell for sure. Sometimes, fitness and health coaches give up on the subject and just say: *It differs according to what works with a person's body.*

Is there any truth to this claim? The debate about carbs is similar. Looking back at the history of dieting, there is a constant shift — back and forth — between promoting the consumption of carbs and the total elimination of carbs from one's diet. Have you heard about the *bread diet?* Yes, it did exist early in the 20th century. This diet encouraged women who intended to lose weight to simply survive on bread. And bread is full of carbs!

Later on, one will see the rise of the *high-protein, high-fat diet*, which now de-emphasizes the consumption of carbs. There are many more fad diets that constantly keep an eye out for the consumption of carbs — whether to encourage or to discourage — and even now, after thousands of researches and studies, nobody could still say for sure whether one should avoid carbs or not.

However, one thing is certain: *The human body needs carbs.* Carbs are essential to one's health, regardless of the popular acclaim for low-carb diets or no-carb diets. True, these diets *do* result in weight loss, fat loss, and better health, but there is a *huge compromise* to be made!

The physical need for carbs is debatable, but on a practical level, one can seriously ask: *What is life without carbs?* In theory, one may be able to completely eliminate carbs, but how does this work in reality? For one reason, it is very difficult to sustain a diet without consuming carbs. This is very costly to begin with. A second reason — truly worth defending — is that most of the time, *good food is made of carbs.*

Think about every yummy, satisfying, and delectable food that you can imagine — you bet they're full of carbs! One must indulge in good taste and good food once in a while. This is part of a satisfying lifestyle! Lastly, the consumption of carbs is embedded in human culture such that *one cannot just avoid it.*

To deliberately cut out food groups and live without carbs is, basically, to start a culture of your own. This means saying goodbye to Pizza Fridays, being unable to go out with friends on a food adventure, and being extra-selective when you go to hosted parties and other gatherings. So many cultures also have carbs as their "national food." Rice is a staple food in Asia, and in Western cultures, one sees bread, so many kinds of cheeses, beverages, burritos, and countless food that are more or less grouped under the category of *carbohydrates*.

So why say goodbye to carbs? This book encourages you to taste the good side of life and indulge once in a while. Of course, you will be taught about eating carbs *properly*. How much carbs do you truly need? Why do you need carbs in the first place? How can you become lean and melt fat simply by eating the *proper* amount of carbs?

If you truly love carbs but wish to become lean and melt fat, then this book is certainly written for you. So read on and be enlightened.

Chapter 2: Scrutinizing Carbs

How much do you know about carbs? Have you researched about this controversial food molecule? You do not have to be a chemist or a dietician to know the truth about carbs. However, there are basic truths — mostly general knowledge — about carbs that you do need to know. These are very easy to understand, and it is most likely that you have encountered this in your high school education. The truth about carbs is not at all elusive!

Truth 1: Carbs are sources of energy. This is an indisputable claim. To acquire energy for everyday needs, people need carbs. Carbohydrates are the primary source of energy especially for vigorous activities such as running, hiking, swimming, and other sports. Athletes cannot possibly — or with much difficulty — adopt a no-carb diet. To do so would make them incompetent in their sport and have a significant disadvantage from those who add carbs as part of their diet.

But what about bodybuilders who survive on meat? It is true that these people exist, to the envy or insecurity of many. The bulk of their muscles and significant strength make everyone think that it is possible to live without carbs at all.

Is this true? Look at the big picture: What activities do these people engage in? Weightlifting and running are two different things, in the same way that strength and speed are two different things. The activities that these people engage in *do not require* a significant amount of carbs. Besides, even foods in the category of protein *do* contain an amount of carbohydrates. Unless you live on protein shakes and amino acid pills, you cannot certainly achieve a "no-carb" diet. This diet is a myth, or an unsustainable reality.

Truth 2: Carbs are found in every food group. This has been mentioned previously, but it is important to elaborate the point further. Unless you're talking about coffee or water, there will always be some amount of carbs involved. Fruits have carbs, bread has carbs, vegetables have carbs, and meat has carbs. There is no escape from carbs. There are, however, varying amounts of carbs in these foods — and you will learn about this later. It is important to know the amount of carbs in a certain food type, so that it will be easier for you to track your consumption.

Truth 3: Carbs do not turn into fat. This is a common — and annoying — misconception about carbohydrates. When you see someone eating a slice of cake or finishing a pint of ice cream, you feel bad for the person because you think that the calories from carbohydrates become *converted* into fat. There has never been a claim more wrong than this! When you consume carbohydrates, they are burned and are used to produce *energy*. They do not become fat the moment that they are consumed.

Having a *carbohydrate surplus* is a different story, though. This is the part when carbs *do* turn into fat, but this happens because there is a *surplus* of carbohydrates. If the body cannot burn carbs into energy, they become stored for future use as *fat*. As a matter of fact, even *protein surplus* can make you fat. A person can accumulate fat from *any food category*, as long as there is a *surplus*.

Truth 4: Carbs are good for you. Believe it or not, your body gets a lot of benefit from carbohydrate consumption. They increase your energy levels and make sure that you do not feel lethargic during the day. True, people on a very low-carb diet still feel energetic, but that is because their bodies *synthesize other compounds to make up for the lack of carbohydrate consumption.* These compounds either involve muscle or fat. With a very low-carb diet, a person may lose an amount of fat, but at the same time, lose muscle. Nobody wants to lose muscle! If you want to stay lean, you would need to maintain a good balance between fat and muscle. And remember: Too little fat is not good for your body!

Keep these three truths in mind whenever you consume carbs, or whenever someone discourages you to consume carbs. In the next chapter, you will know *exactly* how much carbs do you need so you can get an idea of eating the "proper" amount of carbs.

Chapter 3: How Much Carbs Do You Need?

Since it is now established that one need carbs in order to survive, the next big question is: *How much carbs exactly does one need?*

This is a very simple question. However, the process toward answering the question is a little more complex. It is not *difficult* to find out how much carbs are needed, but there are a lot of factors to consider. You will have to consider these factors one by one, and it is up you to figure out — with the guidance of this book — the proper amount of carbs that you need to achieve your specific goals.

Lose weight or maintain weight? You must know what your goals are. Do you intend to build muscle while losing fat, a.k.a. *body recomposition?* Do you intend to lose fat only and look lean? Are you content with your weight and simply want to maintain it? Be clear with what you want.

The ideal carb intake, in simple terms, is the *amount that you have to intake after your protein and fat consumptions have been factored in.* Yes, if you do intend to count your calories, you should also be aware of what your protein and fat intakes are.

Complicated? Don't worry! There are countless dieting apps that you can use to figure out exactly how much protein, carbs, and fat are in a certain food type. You may use these apps or take matters into your own hands by doing research, reading food labels, and making calculations.

Isn't this process exhausting and time-consuming? You will have to make manual calculations *until* you have figured out exactly the amount and kinds of food that you need. In this case, the calculation becomes *instinctive*, and you wouldn't have to always use the calculator and review your every food intake for the day.

Know your caloric needs. Go online and find an effective, ideal calorie intake calculator. Your caloric needs would depend on your weight, height, and activity level. You will get an approximation of the calories that you need, which will range from 1,200 to 3,000.

To lose weight, it is safe to cut 500 to 1000 calories from your caloric needs. The amount that you intend to trim depends on how fast you intend to lose weight. The same is true for weight gain, in case you want to add muscle.

Make the calculation. This is easier than you think. For this part, you would have to come up with a good food plan according to your needs and the food available to you. Simplify the process and follow these steps:

1. After calculating your ideal caloric intake, subtract the amount of carbs that you intend to intake.
   A *moderate* carbohydrate intake has about 400 to 600 calories — this is about 100 to 150 grams. To lose fat, you may want to lessen your carb intake by 50 grams or 200 calories. Count the total amount of carbs (in calories) that you need to consume to achieve your goal. Subtract this from your basic caloric needs.
2. The difference would be the amount of calories that you can consume from protein and fat. You should consume more protein than fat, and remember that protein has *4 calories* per gram, whereas fat as *9 calories* per gram.

If you have trouble making calculations, you may always seek the help of someone who is good at math! Just remember the following formula:

Total caloric intake – Protein intake – Fat intake = Carb intake

This formula is designed to make sure that you do not consume any carbohydrate surplus.

Find out the foods that you can consume from your targeted caloric intake. This is very easy, but then again, you would have to use math and some basic research. Again, don't be discouraged, because you will soon learn this by heart!

When learning a new recipe, make sure to check for the grams of carbohydrates or carbohydrate calories that are involved. Be consistent with your calculations and make sure that you do not consume more calories than your limit. This is the best way to limit your carb intake, instead of simply relying on *guilt* — the topic of the next chapter.

Chapter 4: Being Carb-Sensitive

After following the steps from the last chapter, you will see a figure that you would need to follow and keep in mind. Whether this is 1,200 calories or 2,500 calories, you would have to take it seriously. Can you do this? You certainly can! All you need is *discipline*.

There are so many food items to choose from, with varying amounts of carbs and calories. You may find yourself confused about how to plan your food, or rather *excited* by the prospect of getting your *rewards* and tickets to *indulgence* once in a while. You may even be inclined to learn new recipes and discover food that will fit your caloric goals!

In this chapter, you will get to choose and adopt a proper mindset in order to shape your discipline toward food. But remember, these are only guidelines — only you, yourself, could find the discipline that will work for you.

What levels of change do you have to make? You should know how far the leap is before taking it. Remember, you do not need to be too hard on yourself. Dieting is a lifestyle change, and everyone knows how lifestyle changes can cause a significant deal of stress. Heck, stress causes fat gain in most people! If you're the type to eat everything on the table, you may need to take a huge leap.

You should be prepared to make the leap and have the right *momentum* before taking the jump. Visualize the extent of changes that you need to make. Make sure that you have completely *made up* your mind about this lifestyle choice. *Always remind yourself of your motivations*. Remember: You can do it. People have lost unbelievable amounts of weight after varying periods of time. Do not pressure yourself. Losing weight slowly but surely is a medical advice.

Redefine your indulgence and your rewards. Nothing feels better than finishing a big burger oozing with cheese and eating unlimited numbers of cupcakes after a hard day's work. It is a good thing to reward yourself, but rewards only become rewards if they are given due to the achievement of something *worthwhile*. If you reward yourself every day, you are making the concept of rewards very fluid. It becomes more of a lifestyle than a reward system.

Realize that indulgence has to be *earned*. If you are not into the concept of rewards, then think of indulging as a way to give yourself a break or to breathe from the stress of life. Of course, you cannot do this on a frequent basis. You should be clear on what should be regular in your food list and what should not. And since the subject is *carbs*, you would have to be aware of the amount of carbs that are considered on the "reward" or "indulgence" level. If you love pizza, then make sure that you have Pizza Fridays only twice or thrice a month — not twice or thrice a week. This method will also make you learn how to *appreciate* food better.

Develop a good relationship with food. Food is your friend. Do not use food as an escape or a way to get rid of the negativities in your life. Treat it with respect. Would you use your friends for the sake of moving on from the stress of daily work? You may do so, but you would have to do it in a way that you all benefit and nobody feels used. Never open a bag of chips just because you are feeling lonely, in the same way that you do not call your friend just because you need someone to talk to, or for other selfish reasons. See food as an anchor that provides you with life and the energy to live. Never abuse it: Eat food with respect for the food itself and, most especially, yourself.

Chapter 5: The "Ideal Carb" Diet Regime

Where should you get your source of carbs?

You should remember that carbs — just like calories — are not all the same. For example, consuming 400 calories of peanut butter is not the same as consuming 400 calories of salad. First of all, these two vary in *volume* or amount (There are less calories in a cup of fruit in comparison to a cup of peanut butter!) and they vary in components such as protein, carbohydrates, and fat. Therefore, you should avoid counting calories alone and relying on figures. You should know what composes a calorie. The same is true with carbohydrates — a carbohydrate is not always just one carbohydrate.

There are many different types of carbs with varying molecular complexities, but there is no need to dwell on that. To keep matters simple and short, what you need to know is that there are *good sources* of carbs and there are *bad sources* of carbs.

Good sources of carbs include natural, unprocessed food. You may be familiar with them. Potatoes, rice, grains, and other naturally occurring food — processed minimally — are good sources of carbohydrates. Your staple food for carbohydrates should come from these types of food. Don't worry about the lack of diversity in terms of the dishes and meals that you can have. You will be surprised with the variety of recipes that you can make with unprocessed food!

There is also such as a thing as a *glycemic index*. In layman's terms, this means the amount of sugar in a particular carbohydrate-rich food. Carbohydrates are sugars, basically, but some food types have more sugar than others because of glucose, fructose, and other naturally occurring sugars. For example, in fruits, grapes have a higher glycemic index compared to melons. You should avoid these sugary foods. When consuming your carbohydrates, keep in mind the amount of sugar involved.

A Word On Processed Carbs

Bread, pasta, pastries, and other white carbs are often appraised negatively. A common dieting advice is to avoid "white" carbs, and stick to colored ones such as those found in potatoes, wheat, and vegetables. This dieting advice is valid to a large extent, since non-white carbs are indeed nutritious — by virtue of the fact that they are not processed.

But if you cannot avoid white carbs completely, make sure that you consume them after a heavy physical activity, particularly after working out. During this time, the body burns more calories, and the calories that are stored in white carbs are better synthesized.

Chapter 6: Sustaining Your Fat Loss

After weeks of eating the right amount of carbs — coupled with a calorie deficit, if you intend to lose weight — you will indeed melt fat. This is a scientific process! With a heavier weight, your body would require more calories and carbohydrates to produce the energy that you need for your weight, age, and activity level. If you cut down on your calorie intake, especially your carbohydrate intake, you will definitely have nothing else to melt but *fat*. Your body will not burn muscle if you consume the right amount of proteins and if you meet the caloric needs that your body truly needs.

To make sure that you stay lean, the best advice is to continue following your diet regime, coupled with exercise. Never lose your discipline. Good exercise and a perfect diet make a good combo. Besides, exercising makes you burn more calories, giving ample space for you to eat more of the food that you truly love. This makes room for rewards, indulgence, and the excitement for baking that cake or pastry for your simple enjoyment.

The truth about fat loss and weight loss is that often, it is more difficult to *maintain* the fat loss than to trigger the fat loss itself. You have probably seen this with many people, who slowly gain pounds after weight loss, until they have found themselves reverting back to their original weight. Achieving weight loss after you have re-gained the fat is more difficult, because at this point, your body will start to cling to the fat.

The most important thing to remember about eating the right amount of carbs is being able to incorporate it into your lifestyle. Once you are able to eat the right amount of carbs *by heart*, you will more or less sustain your weight loss, with a fluctuation of one or two pounds. True, in the beginning you will have to make tedious calculations and take huge leaps in terms of fixing your lifestyle. The most important key here is to never lose your motivation. Through time, you will realize that eating the proper amount of carbs is just the same as living a healthy lifestyle and focusing on your well-being.

The most effective way to stay lean and keep the weight off is to always have the proper mindset, coupled with discipline and action. In the previous chapters, you have been taught everything that you needed to learn — the nature of carbs, the right consumption, and how to choose food that will make your dieting possible.

Now, the achievement of fat loss, a great figure, and a good-looking body (with or without clothes!) is all in your hands.

Conclusion

I hope you were able to receive a lot of value from this book.

Low-carbohydrate diets are excellent.

They have been shown to be effective against some of the world's biggest health problems.

This includes obesity, diabetes, metabolic syndrome and a few others.

More than 20 randomized controlled trials have been conducted in the past 10 years.

These studies consistently show that low-carb diets cause more weight loss and greater improvements in health markers, compared to the standard low-fat diet.

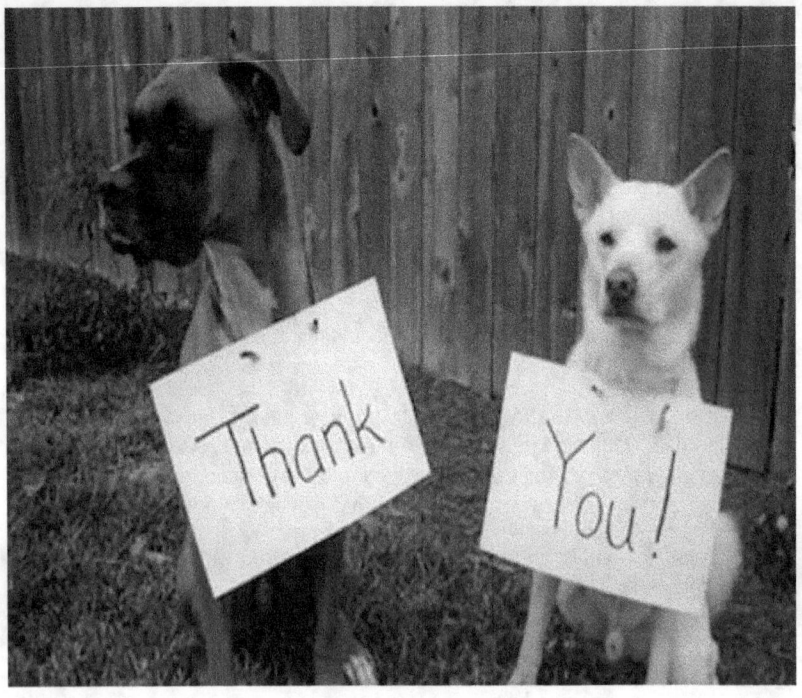

Finally, if you enjoyed this book, then I'd like to ask you for a favor, would you be kind enough to leave a review for this book on Amazon? It'd be greatly appreciated!

Click here to leave a review for this book on Amazon!

Thank you and good luck!